How to Start Your Own Day-Spa

LEONARD PAYNE

DEDICATION

To all those who assist and make life smoother

CONTENTS

ACKNOWLEDGMENTS

To all who make life easier and smoother – Thank You
The mistakes are all mine

1
INTRODUCTION

The day spa industry is booming and you can find great success in this field. There is vast opportunity in this industry and it promises an outstanding future. There are many considerations to make before opening your day spa beginning with the benefits.

The economy has its ups and downs and it may seem unlikely that the day spa industry would hold up in the midst of economic dismay. However, this service industry continues to flourish during hard times. It does exceedingly well when the economy is booming.

There is good reason for the success of this realm of the service sector. A trip to a day spa is relatively inexpensive compared to high-ticket items like an SUV or the latest technological gadgets. Customers enjoy a relaxing experience that leaves them feeling and looking terrific.

The day spa experience helps to ease stress, which is of the utmost importance in today's society. Many people recognize the benefit of taking time to relax and enjoy special treatment. The services offered by many of these organizations are conducive to stress relief.

Health is another issue to consider. Customers are addressing some of their health issues when they enter a day spa. Services like massages and facials can reduce stress, which has significant health benefits. Clients leave with a healthy glow.

Looks are very important to many people. Good health and good looks are closely linked. Some day spa services are designed to help customers look their best. Treatments like body wraps can take inches off in just a single visit and facial treatments can take years off a person's face.

Baby boomers are also a significant factor in your decision to open a day spa. This generation is apt to use the services offered by spas, especially since they are conducive to good health. Many baby boomers are willing to invest in services that will make them look and feel better.

Opening a day spa may be a good choice for you because this type of service is nearly impossible to reproduce at home. People really can't have a "home spa" without investing considerable money. It is more affordable for customers to visit a spa rather than purchase the supplies necessary to create one at home.

The people who work in day spas are trained professionals that have special skills that are difficult to replicate. Consumers can save time by visiting an establishment that offers a variety of different services conducted by skilled professionals in a one-stop facility rather than making appointments all over town.

The day spa industry is lush, promising great success if you plan well. Your business plan and smart marketing approach can help you achieve your goals.

2
WHY A DAY SPA MIGHT BE THE BUSINESS FOR YOU

The very notion of opening a day spa may be appealing to you. This business is ideal for a service-minded individual who likes recognition for dedication and hard work. When you open an establishment like this, you have the unique opportunity to improve the quality of life for your customers. They enjoy the services and they leave refreshed and feeling better about themselves.

Day spas can be lucrative if you have good business sense. If you have outstanding management and organizational skills, you can opt to run the business yourself. You can also opt to hire a spa manager to help you keep your hectic schedule under control.

There are many things to think about when entering such a venture and your general interest in the day spa business is a first step. Interest is not enough to move you towards achieving success. You also must learn about the industry as well.

A LOOK AT THE INDUSTRY

Years ago, spas were reserved for the very wealthy or for people who wanted to lose weight. These facilities were quite popular during the 19th century. The Kellog brothers operated a health spa that focused on healthy habits and a variety of treatments that were designed to help improve the clients' overall health.

Proper diet was among the interventions used at the Kellog spa. The Kellog brothers invented Corn Flakes to promote a fiber-rich diet to their members. The cereal made an impact on the mass market in 1906 and it continues to be a popular, healthy choice for breakfast.

Spas typically focused on helping people improve or maintain their health. They have grown to address nearly every aspect of human wellness including spiritual and emotional. Today's services offer whole body treatments and deep relaxation strategies that are ideal for overall health.

The development of the day spa helped to make these healthful and relaxing services available to the public. These facilities are appealing to a wide spectrum of customers, each looking for various services and products.

Consumers no longer have to go to destination spas to receive outstanding treatments for a reasonable price. There are elements of fashion, retail, health issues and aesthetic treatments in these facilities. There is even a hint of interior design as well.

The wellness movement is the driving force behind the day spa trade. People of various ages and backgrounds are now drawn to these facilities. The day spa is convenient because the consumer is only in the spa for as long as it takes to complete the treatment.

Much of the population looks at regular visits to the day spa as a requirement for good health rather than a luxury. Consumers no longer have to wait for a vacation or special weekend getaway to enjoy the treatments. These facilities have become an integral part of healthy interventions.

People are frequenting day spas on a regular basis and talented professionals are entering spa-inspired vocations as well. Many skilled people have the knowledge and expertise to help you deliver some of the most popular services offered by the industry.

There are many services to offer and pairing the right services with the right employees can make all the difference in your endeavor. Traditional services available in the day spa industry include:

- Massages
- Facials
- Waxing
- Manicures and Pedicures
- Hydrotherapies
- Steam rooms
- Exercise Equipment

There are also many newer services to consider as well:

- Aromatherapy
- Hot Rock Massage
- Green Spa Treatments
- Personal Trainers
- Body Wraps
- Salt Glows
- Gemstone Treatments
- Detoxification

The lists are not comprehensive. You can include many other services as well. Some day spa owners offer limousine rides and champagne. Others offer hair salon services. The population close to your facility's location should dictate which services you choose.

THE MARKETS WHERE DAY SPAS FLOURISH

Wide ranges of people are very interested in spa treatments because there is such an undercurrent of holistic, natural and organic components in them. People are drawn to day spas since they relate to natural health remedies and healthy habits.

Day spas are particularly appealing because they are very affordable compared to destination spas. People from various economic backgrounds can afford regular visits to day spas. Making them accessible to the massive audience can be a very lucrative decision.

There is a great demand for convenient day spa services and it is crucial that you choose your featured treatments according to the demographics in your region. There may be a great demand for services that promote weight loss but little interest in hydrotherapies in your area.

Many people are in the market for stress relief. Some spa treatments are very effective in helping people relax. This is important to people concerned about physical and mental health problems that can result from excessive stress.

The spa industry has many standard treatments that continue to be popular generation after generation. This industry also has many trends that peak in popularity. Some current trends include detoxification and gemstone massage. It is necessary to keep up with the trends by attending day spa conferences and studying the most recent development in the market.

<u>3</u>
<u>MARKET RESEARCH MATTERS</u>

Market research is an integral part of your day spa's success. It is imperative that you carefully consider the population near your business. You may be very interested in caviar facials but if your potential clients are not, the treatment is not going to have a great impact.

Your potential customers are your day spa's potential. One of the most important aspects of developing a plan to open a new business is to become familiar with the demographics in your area. This is a basic concept in the law of supply and demand.

KNOW YOUR DEMOGRAPHICS

Getting to know your demographics requires some footwork but it pays off in the end. A great approach is to get a membership to the International Spa

Association (ISPA). This organization publishes a report that outlines habits of spa users. The Spa Users Report is available to members at half the cost than for nonmembers.

The general demographics indicate that the typical spa user is married and has a college education. Typically, they come from households that do not have children under the age of eighteen and they are employed full time. They are generally in their early to mid forties.

The vast majority of spa goers are women. Only about twenty percent of the spa users are men. Household income for the typical client is about $95,000 dollars annually. These demographics can give you an idea of which services are best to cater to your specific population.

Considering the general demographics, you would most likely choose treatments that have anti-aging elements as well as stress-reducing services. Since many of the people work at least part time, you will have to accommodate them by being available during the evening and on weekends.

Men do make up a portion of the spa-goers so it is helpful to have some services for this population. Current trends suggest that couples are taking trips to day spas together. Knowing this, you can sell a couple package to one of your female clients in hopes of getting her partner's business as well.

The community that you choose is important, too. Conservative towns will have different wants and needs than liberal ones. Some regions opt for treatments that make them look younger while others focus on health as their primary issue of concern.

Your advertising, atmosphere, services and hours of operation depend heavily on the demographics. A day spa is a service industry. The customer is the most important factor.

UNDERSTAND WHAT YOUR POTENTIAL CLIENTS REALLY WANT

No matter what the service or product, people want value. This doesn't mean that they want something for next to nothing. They just want to have a great experience that doesn't leave them with buyer's remorse.

The very notion of a day spa conjures images of pampering and luxury. Many people are not comfortable making regular visits to a spa because they may feel guilty for being so extravagant. It is helpful if you express how beneficial these visits are to the consumer's overall wellbeing.

Package deals are perfect because they allow you to sell more treatments at a lower cost. The client saves money while enjoying stress-reducing, healthful treatments. The package deals should contain services that complement each other.

Consider wet services versus dry services. You have studied the demographics so you know whether the population is comfortable with wet treatments. Hydrotherapy requires the customer to remove clothing. Some people may shy away from these services.

A package could include a wet service like a mineral soak followed by a body wrap. The services would be complemented by a facial and makeup application. Plan your packages according to how long each activity takes.

If you are going to embrace the package deals in full force, you might want to include a light lunch or snack. Some may want to include champagne or sparkling juice. The packages may take three to five hours to complete in some cases.

Package deals make wonderful gifts and they are perfect for bridal parties and birthdays. You could include limousine services arranged with a local limo company depending on the season and the demographics.

The economy is a factor to consider as well. Research your potential customers' economic base in order to decide what variety of services and specials to consider. The city's economic development office should be able to give you an idea of how strong the region's industry is. You want to forgo gemstone massages in a blue-collar town that is in the throes of economic hardship.

PUT IT ALL TOGETHER

Your day spa should embrace the wants and needs of the customers in your vicinity. The basic law of supply and demand suggests that you should provide services that are in demand but may be lacking in your region. The best place to begin is to consider your demographics and the most recent developments in the spa industry.

Get to know the current trends in Hollywood and New York. Follow popular programs and talk shows to get an idea of what your target market wants.

Measure whether hot new trends are necessary or whether you should stick to the basics.

Most of your decisions will fall into place once you have a grasp of your target market. Your potential customers will influence your package deals and they will help you decide which services are right for the day spa.

<u>4</u>
<u>MAKING THE INITIAL PLAN</u>

Your initial plan is crucial to the success of your day spa business. There are three major components to the plan to consider beginning with your target audience. This factor will help you decide which type of spa is right for you and your clientele. You also can use the target audience and the services you choose to determine your price points.

Demographic information and market research helps you determine who to target as your customer base. The current trends may influence your potential clients or they may prefer traditional spa services. Pricing depends on the services and the economy in your region.

PICK YOUR TARGET AUDIENCE

Your market research and exploration of the demographics in your region offer valuable information about your target audience. This is one of the most important aspects of your research. You can have outstanding products and services but your client base has to be interested in them for your spa business to succeed.

The demographic profile is all-important in your research. This information determines which services you are going to choose. Your hours of operation depend heavily on the availability of your clientele. If your spa is located in an area that has a high population of working moms, your hours of operation have to accommodate their hectic schedules in order to succeed.

Your day spa needs to accommodate the size of the potential market. You may find that a small facility that accommodates a two or three clients at a time works well for your demographic area. It is always a good idea to design your spa to feel comfortable to the visitors.

A cavernous space that is suitable for fifty people isn't going to provide the intimate atmosphere required in many situations. The size of the size of the potential market will help determine the design of the layout. You may find that your facility requires an ample waiting area that offers a relaxing atmosphere.

Your demographics and market research can help you determine the number of potential clients that used spa services in the past. It helps to know which services they used and whether these can be included in your plan. This information is readily available if you purchase a formerly established day spa.

Some prospects have never been to a spa and you may be able to tap into this resource by introducing one or two innovative services or through a clever advertising campaign. You have to determine whether the population falls into a demographic that typically uses spa services in other regions.

Profiling the potential clients can involve examining your competition. This includes day spas that were in service and have closed their doors. What services did these establishments offer? Why are they no longer in business? Is there a demand for the same type of spa that closed its doors? What can you change to make your day spa more successful?

When you examine your competition, you can also look at day spas that are currently open in the general area. Take time to visit your competition. What would you change? What really worked? Are there services that you can offer that they don't?

Consider the population's general health concerns. You can cater to your potential clients by integrating services that help reduce blood pressure or assist weight loss or any number of other treatments that are healthful.

Relaxation is a primary factor that can help alleviate many conditions.

Health issues are strong motivators and there are other reasons that people visit day spas to consider. Prospective clients may be motivated to reduce stress in their lives by using spa facilities. Others may be motivated to remove toxins from their bodies.

Weight loss is a very popular reason that many customers are interested in day spa treatments. This is a powerful motivator because it addresses several issues. Losing weight improves health, appearance and overall self-esteem. Different people seek treatments to address weight issues for various reasons, giving them universal appeal.

Many potential customers want to improve their appearance and you can provide the services they need. Your target audience may be entering middle age or they may be younger clients who want Hollywood-inspired treatments.

WHAT TYPE OF SPA IS RIGHT FOR YOU AND YOUR CLIENTELE?

The market analysis and demographic research helps you establish what type of spa is right for you and your clientele. You are an integral part of the mix as well. Considering that the market is very promising and many services are appealing to your potential clients, you have chosen an excellent venue.

Other entrepreneurs are well aware of this and there can be a lot of competition to consider. In order to be successful in your venture, you should consider your own personal tastes and personality when developing your plan. This is a wonderful approach to creating a unique and genuine atmosphere.

Consider creating a niche for your day spa that makes your business stand out from the others. Niches are interesting because they address a demand that is not in the mainstream. Having a specialty service that puts a new spin on a well-established idea is a great approach.

Your unique personality and style can help you create a niche for your spa business. Development involves creating a mission that is inspired by your personal vision. This vision should take current market trends and the demographics into consideration.

There are two important elements to developing your niche. You should have a purpose and you should be able to communicate this purpose to your target audience. This approach helps you stay focused in the face of distracting services and products.

For example, if your spa's purpose is to help people create healthy lifestyles, you should cater your services and products to this end. Adding nail services, fingernail polish and accessories into mix distracts your from your primary purpose. A health day spa that offers this type of services is not in tune with your niche.

Instead, it is better to focus on your purpose by including products and services that suit your niche. The health-inspired day spa would focus on detoxification, relaxation, nutrition, and weight control. This purpose needs to be very clear to your potential clients.

Effectively communicating your purpose helps potential customers recognize your niche. Communication also helps them recognize how some of the services benefit them. You can also point out the complementary benefits as well, like health and attractiveness go hand-in-hand.

It can be very tempting try to offer every service possible in the day spa industry but this approach is not realistic or feasible. Study the demographics and the market to determine which services to offer your clientele.

SELECT YOUR PRICE POINTS

Price points can be tricky, especially when you consider all of the overhead you face when opening a day spa. A delicate balance to consider includes your expenses and the demographic information you have collected about your target service area. Setting prices too high will deter many clients and setting prices too low puts your business at risk.

The services you select should suit the demographics. This helps make setting your prices much easier. High-end day spa services are typically reserved for areas that have clientele that can afford them. Package deals are wonderful sellers that are cost effective for you to create and can help boost sales while offer value.

You can effectively create value packages of goods and services when you consider four factors: overhead, inventory, labor and profit. These elements require careful consideration and they stem out of the services that you choose based on the demographics.

Overhead costs include the cost of operation that involves your location. Common overhead costs include leases or mortgages, utilities, phone access, and similar and the like. These components are very important to the success of your company.

Your inventory should be well stocked and you need to consider how often you need to restock. Consider the purchase price of equipment as well as the cost of maintaining it. Tools are not one-time purchases, either. Make room for replacement tools and equipment if the need arises.

You will need employees who are well trained and professional. In order to attract and keep the right professionals you need to offer competitive wages. Your demographics and market analysis help you choose which skilled workers to choose and whether you will need a receptionist, manager or other administrative assistants.

Figure salaries according to hourly productivity and prevailing wages in your demographic area. Don't forget your salary when figuring employee salaries. Hourly wages are generally easier to establish and maintain than yearly salaries in the service industry.

Overhead is typically between forty and fifty percent of the inventory and labor costs. Add all of your inventory and labor costs to determine how much your overhead expense should be. For example, if you add your labor and supply costs for a year to come up with a figure of $200,000, your estimated overhead are estimated between $80,000 and $100,000.

Profit is another consideration to make in your price points. In the current industry, you can expect a profit between eleven and fifteen percent after taxes. This figure depends on how much you charge for services and how much business you attract.

Mark-ups on products and services have a great affect on your profit margin. The process of figuring your prices for products and services can be simplified by considering how much you need to make in a year and work back from there.

If you want to make $52,000 for the year, the spa needs to bring in $1,000 dollars each week to get to that figure. If the spa is open fifty hours a week, it has to make $20 an hour to reach the $1,000 per week goal.

Now that you have an hourly rate, you can figure in your profit margin. The average profit margin is between eleven and fifteen percent. If you want to make a thirteen percent profit margin, the salon needs to make an additional $2.60 cents per hour, making the hourly rate $22.60. The extra $2.60 an hour translates into a profit margin of $6,760 by the end of the year.

This is a very simplistic outline but it gives you a general idea of how setting price points work. Setting the prices in your establishment takes some consideration and every faction counts.

<u>5</u>
<u>FLESHING OUT YOUR PLAN</u>

Fleshing out your plan involves more research but this endeavor is fun. Your day spa should be unique and this requires considering the competition. Once you get to know your competition, you are in a great position to develop a unique theme and select products and services for your day spa. Adding extra touches is a valuable part of fleshing out your plan, too.

GET TO KNOW YOUR COMPETITION

Get to know your competition so you can position your business well. The first step is to create a list of relevant competitors near your day spa's location. Develop a basis of competition that includes details about the organization. Take note of the following:

- Location
- Price
- Services

- Products
- Advertising campaigns
- Target audience
- Quality
- Reputation
- Specials and discounts
- Theme

Taking time to visit the competition can help you get a customer's perspective. As you spend time at the day spas, take note of what does and what doesn't work. Did a receptionist greet you or did you have to wait for a frazzled employee to address you?

What would you suggest they change to make their business run smoother? Take note of things that really impressed you and things that made you cringe. Appreciate the setting and the theme. Is the atmosphere relaxing or clinical?

There may be wonderful ideas for you to consider as you flesh out your plan but it is important to remember to emulate the successful aspects of the competition's business, not copy them. Imitation might be the greatest form of flattery but it doesn't make good business sense.

Try a complementary approach when fleshing out your plan. There may be a demand for a service that your competition is missing. Maybe there is something lacking in their ad campaigns. Perhaps you could develop a unique atmosphere that is warm and welcoming when the competition features a cold, clinical setting.

Make comparisons to your vision of the perfect day spa and the places you explore in your research. See what demographic visits these spas, what programs they offer. Are there any special facilities or amenities that really stand out?

Consider exploring competition within a fifty-mile radius. This may seem extreme but these facilities have a lot of information to offer, especially if they are very successful. Consider the client base that visits these sites because the demographics are most likely to be similar within this radius.

PICKING YOUR THEME

Your theme provides you the opportunity to put your unique personality into your endeavor. The first thing you must consider is whether you are building the business from its foundation or purchasing an existing structure. If you are doing the former, you have many considerations to make.

Primarily, it is crucial to hire an architect or construction team that knows about the spa business. The setting should have a flow of energy that is calming and it should be welcoming, especially if you are going to have a wet room.

You may not have control over the design from the ground up so it is important to be able to be flexible with your ideas. Consider some aspects of your day spa. What makes it unusual? What services are you going to offer? How long is the average stay going to be? These questions can help you develop a general idea of how you want to present your business.

One of the most important aspects of your theme is your personal vision. You chose the day spa business for a reason. Consider the purpose of your facility. What do you want to accomplish? Having purpose and vision is important for you create a unique theme.

For example, you might have a great interest in improving the environment. A biodynamic spa may be the right choice for you depending on the demographics in your area. These spas use natural resources to inspire workers and clients to live natural, healthier lives.

The focus is on organic products that are safe for the environment. The staff practices conservation of resources and the entire operation is environmentally responsible. Renewable energy, philanthropic ventures and health are primary elements in the biodynamic facility.

While your vision is very important, your budget is a fundamental consideration. You can create an impressive atmosphere within your budget, especially if your basic services suit the purpose of the day spa. Consider the demographics, the market and the services that appeal to you.

SELECTING YOUR SERVICES

Consider the day spa services that are available. Many of these might appeal to you and they could possibly suit your theme, but they may not fit your budget. Consider how much you can spend and set your priorities according to your personal vision and the theme you have chosen. Following are examples of services to consider.

Massage

Many people think of massages when they think of spas. This service is designed to help promote healing and relaxation and it has much appeal for a wide range of clientele. This treatment manipulates the soft tissue on the body, providing therapeutic help.

Massage services require professional massage therapist. Typically, the treatment requires massage tables and chairs but some facilities use floor mats. The client will require a changing area to prepare for the massage in most cases.

There is a great demand for this service for people who have tension, back and muscular problems. The treatment is very relaxing and some believe that massage therapy as psychological as well as physical benefits.

There are more than eighty different modalities in massage therapy so you could benefit from further research to decide which modalities are suitable for your client base. Another consideration to make is finding skilled massage therapists who specialize in certain modalities of massage therapy.

Facials

Facials are standard services in day spas. These cosmetic procedures are treats for the skin that provide deep cleansing, exfoliating, toning, steaming, massaging, and moisturizing. Products used in facials include moisturizing cream, lotion, peels, masks and gem-infused products.

These services are an integral part of most day-spa experiences because they are in great demand. Unusual facial products hit the market from time to time. Odd examples include bird excrement, caviar and gemstone facials. Your demographics should determine whether the unusual products will sell at your facility.

Skin Exfoliation

Skin Exfoliation is a procedure that is common in facials but this approach deserves recognition as an independent treatment. This health treatment removes dead cells from the surface of the skin. The procedure is applicable to the face and the body.

The treatment boasts excellent results for customers. New, healthy skin emerges as dead cells are removed. The results are measurable because the skin is noticeably healthy looking and smooth.

There are a few products to consider that exfoliate the skin.

Chemical peels are intense treatments that are mostly used on the face. Some clients may require approaches that are even more intense. Dermabrasion and microderemabrasion use sanding mechanisms to remove dead skin cells in some cases. In most instances, you can expect to use abrasive cloths or micro-bead face scrubs to exfoliate.

<u>Waxing</u>

Waxing is another common service that addresses the face and the body. This day spa treatment removes hair by its roots. The process is relatively simple. A licensed cosmetologist or esthetician performs this procedure.

The technician applies a thin layer of hot wax on the specific area that requires hair removal followed by a paper or cloth section. The section is removed quickly, pulling the unwanted hair out by its roots. This process also removes dead skin as well.

This approach is effective in removing hair for up to eight weeks. Many report that the hair grows back thinner and lighter after a waxing treatment. Following are different areas of the body that can use wax spa treatments:

- Legs
- Chest
- Back
- Eyebrows
- Underarms
- Feet
- Bikini

BODY TREATMENTS

Some services are cosmetic in nature and others are therapeutic. Many can be both. Body treatments are nice choices if you plan to have a wet room because they remind customers of luxury spa experiences. Note whether the demographics in your area are drawn to these services.

HOT TUBS, SAUNAS AND MUD BATHS

If your location is close to a workout facility, you might want to include hot tubs and saunas in your list of services. Many people love to unwind using these treatments after a workout. These services are also wonderful if your day spa offers massage therapy.

There is considerable expense to consider when adopting these services into your day spa. Hot tubs, mud baths and saunas demand a substantial investment and they require close maintenance. Make sure that your potential clientele are interested in these services before making a significant investment.

AROMATHERAPY, YOGA AND MEDITATION

Aromatherapy, yoga and mediation appeal to many people in certain demographics. These therapies are somewhat spiritual in nature and can have an eclectic audience. These programs are relatively inexpensive by their simplistic nature but there are some considerations to make.

You will have to hire a professional that is skilled in yoga or meditation instruction. Classes may have to be scheduled and there may be many conflicts if you have a limited number of hours available for these services.

Aromatherapy, on the other hand, is a wonderful treatment across the board because it cost relatively little money and it is very effective. Your investment consists of aromatherapy products, proper lighting and comfortable recliners or applicable seating.

BODY TREATMENTS

Health-conscious and weight-conscious visitors have great interest in body treatments. These include salt scrubs, exfoliation, hot tubs, mud baths, saunas and aromatherapy, among many other treatments. Body wraps are very popular choices to consider.

Body wraps remove excess water weight from the body and they leave skin feeling smooth and soft. This treatment is ideal for clientele who are weight and health-conscious. Body wraps have a detoxifying affect on the body and the customer loses inches along with excess water and toxins.

These treatments use elastic cloths that are pre-soaked in a body wrap mixture of natural herbs that pull fluid and toxins out of the tissue. The cloths are typically wrapped around the torso, arms, legs and neck. The client sees instant results in lost inches and smoother, tighter skin.

BEAUTY SALON SERVICES

The demographics and market research may indicate that there is a demand for salon services in your area. Some day spas offer haircutting and styling as well as hair products. Manicures and pedicures are other popular choices for day spa services that are inspired by beauty salons. Cosmetology in the application of makeup is another option to consider if the demographics point towards an interest in beauty salon services.

There are many more services to consider including steam rooms and personal trainers. The services you select are contingent upon the demographics in your area, availability of trained staff and the spa's theme.

EXTRA TOUCHES THAT MAKE A DIFFERENCE

Little details can go a long way in the day spa industry. Some considerations you can make about the general layout of the spa, the décor and elements help you create an outstanding atmosphere. These considerations should suit your theme.

For example, if you focus on recreating a Roman bathhouse, you would select design elements that relate to the theme. These may include columns, calm water pools and hot tubs. The color scheme could include marble tones and crisp white accents.

A Tuscan theme would include warm, earthy tones and deep purple hues inspired by grapes and wine. The setting could include traditional Tuscan furnishings and rich tapestries that provide depth and interest in the space. These elements should be consistent throughout the spa.

Your theme is the source of design inspiration and you probably already have many ideas spinning through your head. Your décor and accents work together with the layout of the spa to create an atmosphere that clearly communicates your vision and purpose.

Day spas need to be compartmentalized in order for many of the services to be delivered in comfort and privacy. Your theme and purpose are considerable factors in the layout of your spa. Before you can design and decorate, you have to have a clear vision that includes the services you offer.

Take the customer's point of view. Is there a need for a private waiting area? Are consultation rooms necessary? Will products be displayed behind a counter or in the reception area? Your layout can follow any number of patterns.

You may have the reception area in the center with the various service departments branching out from there. Storage should be readily available for workers. If the inventory stock is kept in the basement or in the very back of the building, there should be a space for supplies for quick access in a logical place.

Services and supplies are considerable factors in your design but there are many other considerations to make as well. Lighting is among the most important. You want the area to be calm and relaxing so soft lighting is appropriate.

Some services, like waxing, call for bright overhead lighting. Ideally, these lights can be dimmed or turned completely off while alternative soft lighting fills the space. The lighting elements should be in sync with your overall theme.

Fragrance is important, too but this needs to be approached carefully. If you are offering aromatherapy services, you know the significance of fragrances and you also know that some people can't tolerate certain smells. This detail should be light and barely noticeable. Perfume-rich candles and air freshening products can be overbearing.

Music is very important as well. A stone silent day spa can be uncomfortable and cold. Your selection of music should suit your theme, vision and purpose. Different music can be used in different areas of the spa. This is a subtle touch but this detail should not be overlooked

Use your vision to develop the details that inspire you. Consider striking accents in competitors' spas and use them as a source of encouragement. Your day spa can address every sense, completely immersing your clients in a relaxing, enjoyable experience.

<u>6</u>
<u>ESTIMATE YOUR NEEDS</u>

You can benefit from estimating your needs as you flesh out your day spa plans. This is an integral part of developing a business plan that really works. It can help you keep focus on which services and products are right for your endeavor. Your supplies and staffing needs are of the utmost importance as you make your plans.

EQUIPMENT YOU MIGHT NEED

There are many things to think about as you flesh out your plans and among the most important is the equipment you might need. Your features may require special tools and furnishings in order to provide proper service to your spa guests. There are some considerations to make as you create your approach.

Your facility has to have enough room to accommodate special equipment like furnishings and if you are going to carry products to sell, there needs to be an attractive display area. Ideally, these products are arranged in areas that are accessible to guest rather than stored back behind a counter.

Divide your equipment into several categories as you see fit. For example, you might arrange your list according to services or type of equipment. Your organization can help you stay focused and in control.

Products and tools are plentiful in this industry. Many details need to be considered. Following is a sample list of common products that you may need. Your list will vary according to the specific services that you offer.

Basic Items:

- Cotton balls, swabs and rolls
- Sponges
- Tissues
- Gowns or cover-ups
- Headbands or head covers

- Gauze
- Towels
- Clean sheets
- Makeup trays
- Supply trolleys
- Bobby pins and safety pins
- Scissors, clippers, shavers, scalpels
- Applicators
- Elastic bandages

<u>Products:</u>

- Lotions
- Creams
- Cleansers
- Exfoliating, chemical peels, microdermabrasion
- Facial masks
- Astringent
- Antiseptic
- Soaps, body washes
- Herbs
- Shampoo
- Massage oil

- Aromatherapy candles, oils and creams
- Sun block
- Hand sanitizers

<u>Equipment:</u>

- Facial bed or chair
- Facial massager
- Massage table or chair
- Vibrating body massager
- Orthopedic pillow
- Hot tub, sauna, steam room equipment
- Wax heaters
- Paraffin wax receptacles

These lists are in no way comprehensive but they give you a general idea of the type of equipment you may need. Various services will require different products, supplies and equipment.

ANTICIPATE STAFFING NEEDS

Staffing needs is a very important consideration as well. This subject can be tricky but you can begin organizing by considering the services your day spa will offer. Some of these services require trained, licensed professionals so your staffing needs are quite specific in many instances.

Scheduling is an issue that you develop during the operations stage of your plan. As for now, you can simply concentrate on whom you will hire and whether full-time or part-time employees will be necessary. There are other things to consider like staff employees and independent contractors.

No matter what, you will need core employees to help you run your facility. Begin by considering your hours of operation. Will your day spa offer services seven days a week? Will it be open 50 hours or 100 hours a week? Longer hours require more staff.

Consider how you will function in the business. Are you going to be a hand-on operator that greets clientele, answers phones and keeps inventory? Or are you going to take care of administration duties at the highest level and hire people to address the details and duties.

There are general guidelines in staffing a business to follow. Remember that payroll is going to be your most costly expense in operating your business. The right staff members can make all the difference in the success of your venture. Insufficient pay and lack of hours can drive qualified applicants away.

You have three basic types of employees to consider. Core employees offer help full-time. They typically receive wages and benefits. Part-time employees are ideal for busy times of the week. They earn wages and you may include benefits.

On-call staff includes independent contractors. These professionals are subcontractors who pay you to use your facility while earning money for their trade. You may know a fantastic yoga instructor that is willing to offer classes and instruction on a regular basis.

Check with the demographic area and competition to find out the prevailing wage for services and employees in the day spa industry. These helpful entities can make or break your business. Following are typical jobs employees fill.

- **Managers**

  Managers can help you stay organized by taking care of paperwork, scheduling, purchasing and keeping records. This employee is invaluable if you have a large, successful establishment.

- **Cosmetologist nail technicians or hair stylists**

  These can offer services to your customers. Many day spas choose to adopt services like hair cutting and styling and makeup application. These tasks require talented professionals.

- **Spa assistants**

  Spa assistants can keep stock readily available for technicians and therapists. They can make sure music is playing appropriately and they can help create a clean, comfortable atmosphere. Small tasks like folding towels and gathering necessary equipment and tools can help your day spa run smoothly.

- **Receptionists**

Receptionists greet customers and help them check in and out of the day spa. They answer phones, book appointments and give directions to the facility. Some organizations have managers take on these tasks but you may opt for a receptionist if your business is particularly busy.

- **Aestheticians**

Aestheticians offer a myriad of services that are integral to day spas. These licensed professionals provide waxing, facial, massage and body treatments.

- **Massage therapists**

Massage therapists are trained to provide massage services that are beyond the aesthetician's abilities. Therapists must have massage therapy licenses in most states.

- **Independent contractors**

  These people are not on your payroll but they can provide exceptional services that are in great demand. These professionals are ideal for fad treatments or special events. Sometimes a customer will request a service that requires a subcontractor to fulfill.

Your staff is the heart of your business. Consider the services and hours of operation in order to determine which professionals you should hire on full-time, part-time or as subcontractors.

PULLING IT OFF EVEN IF YOU DON'T HAVE EXPERIENCE

Your purpose and vision are motivating forces behind your day spa business but these alone are not enough to help you succeed. It helps to have the right personnel at your side to make the system work. If you have little experience you may want to hire a consultant to help you sort through the details.

A consultant can serve as a valuable guide who can help you by conducting the necessary market research and studying trends. This individual helps you determine your staffing needs, budget and the services that are right for you and your clientele. The consultant also helps you choose equipment and products.

Check the consultant's references in addition to her portfolio. Design skills are not the only factors to consider so don't be swayed by an impressive presentation that focuses on design elements but never addresses equipment, employees or market research.

Begin with a consultation before making your plan and research the fees the consultant will charge. You can expect to pay between 80 and 500 dollars an hour. In some cases, consultants charge more. The billing terms need to be clear as well.

A consultant may be a significant investment but you can benefit greatly from consulting with a professional if you have no experience. This independent contractor can save you a lot of money in the end.

7
CREATE A BUSINESS PLAN THAT SELLS

Your business plan is the heart of your vision and purpose. It is crucial that you create a plan that effectively communicates your intentions and one that provides a clear picture of what your day spa will offer. Potential investors have to use this plan to determine if your endeavor is a good investment or not.

INFORMATION YOU NEED TO INCLUDE

Your business plan needs to include a healthy amount of information. However, you need to keep the plan succinct and to the point. Unnecessary, confusing details can take away from your project. The plan should include the following information to be effective.

- A detailed financial projection that clearly demonstrates how investors will make money is of the utmost importance
- Detailed information about the projected investor's return of investment
- Projection of how the business will perform over a specific amount of time.
- Gross Sales projection
- Net profit projection
- Best and worst case scenarios
- Organizational structure of the business
- Trends and services
- Target market base
- Ad campaigns
- How you will get sales

Your business plan should follow guidelines that can help communicate how your day spa will generate the necessary business to create a profit.

These include the following:

- Location

- Resources

- Ability to carry out the plan

- Advantages of the products

- The current market trends

- Demographics

- Number of employees

- Type of employees

- Services

- Projected cash flow

Make sure to back your plan with resources that exhibit your research efforts. Include information found in magazines, newspapers and online resources. Professional cited should include government agencies, economists and successful spa moguls. Include copies of your resources and documents to assure that the information is credible.

FUNDING OPTIONS THAT WORK

Getting enough money to get your day spa business started can be stressful but you do have options to consider. Your business plan is an extremely important factor in whether you will get the necessary funding. You can approach a few venues that can help you succeed.

A traditional source of business funding is the Small Business Association (SBA). This is the ultimate resource for you to consider because this organization is well established and it offers impressive funding options for you to consider. The SBA is ideal if you are starting your first business or just getting a new endeavor off the ground.

Conventional bank loans are also wonderful resources for you to consider. If you establish your business as a Limited Liability Company (LLC) in your state, your personal finances and your business finances are completely separate. This is a great way to keep your funding organized and concise.

Investors may want to provide funds for future returns. This approach is ideal for large and small ventures. You share part of your revenue with the investors according to the terms of the agreement.

Conventional lending institutions and investors are going to want to see an impressive business plan. It helps if you can demonstrate that you have the experience and knowledge necessary to make your day spa a success. If you don't, you might want to invest in a consultant to help you develop your business plan.

Successful appropriation of funds is a crucial aspect of the proper development of your day spa. You have to consider the costs of operation and your employee needs in this process. The right financial backing can help you work towards creating a day spa that is in tune with your personal vision and purpose.

<u>8</u>
<u>DON'T FORGET THE LEGALITIES</u>

LICENSING AND OTHER ISSUES

Your employees and independent contractors are mostly likely going to need certification through your state's Board of Cosmetology or in massage therapy. In addition, you may want to have employees get certification specific to day spa operations.

The State Board of Cosmetology works to help protect the public by assuring that spas and other similar establishments follow the regulations and licensing practices required by the state. The mission is to keep conditions clean and safe for the public.

Among the certifications available is Certified Spa Supervisor, or CSS. This test assures that the staff member is well versed in spa management practices. The staff member must pass an exam to get CSS accreditation. This is a wonderful accreditation for you to earn as an owner as well.

Cosmetologist, nail technicians and other staff members will have their own respective licensing and accreditation requirements to meet. The conditions vary from state to state. Many employees follow continuing education programs as well.

Massage therapists typically need about 600 hours of training but this number can vary. Many therapists choose to train longer to learn more about the procedures and to improve their credibility.

Most states require licensing or certification. There are also local regulations in many communities to consider as well. After the proper certification and licensing procedures are completed, additional credits need to be earned every few years to maintain certification.

You also need to consider licensing requirements that your state and local government require for spas. Your day spa should meet the hygiene requirements and your equipment will need a viable maintenance schedule.

Establish your day spa as a business. This requires a business license and other certifications required by your state. You might want to establish a Limited Liability Company to ensure that your personal property and finances are completely separate from your day spa's business.

<u>9</u>
<u>LOCATION, LOCATION, LOCATION</u>

Your choice of location should be contingent upon your market research and analysis of the area. This helps you develop a viable business plan because it provides figures that include the actual volume of your potential market. These numbers help you create financial projections and it help you select a prime location for the services that are in demand in your area.

You can use surveys that are available that provide demographics about day spa customers. An example is Claritas. This company takes surveys concerning different aspects of the day spa industry and its customers. This organization evaluates markets, customers and location sites.

If you are using a consultant, you can work to help determine your location as you develop your business plan. This is a great approach if you have no experience in the day spa industry. Loan officials are more likely to recognize a consultant's qualifications while considering your application.

There are different considerations to make that are contingent upon your budget. You might not have enough money to build your day spa from the ground up but you could invest in a standing building. You may find a franchise opportunity of just happen to find a spa that is closing.

You can also opt for a booth rental relationship with an existing spa. The spa's owner allows you to rent the facilities to conduct business. As a renter, you are responsible for all of your own supplies and mode of operation. This makes you an independent contractor in the spa industry.

When you choose your type of business plan, your location sometimes presents itself. However, it is ideal that you conduct the necessary research in order to assure that you find the right place for your business. Consider the following:

- Other retail establishments should be close by

- Ample parking

- Easy access from byway or highway

- Lots of traffic, including pedestrians

- Clean, landscaped surroundings

- Health facilities and gyms

You may know the location that you want to purchase at first glance. However, it is necessary to conduct the research to make sure that this location is going to help your business flourish.

<u>10</u>
<u>PREPARING FOR YOUR OPENING</u>

You have done your market and demographic research. Your business plan is a success. You have found your location and you have the right funding to back you up in your day spa endeavor. Employees are eagerly waiting for the grand opening. This is an exciting time for you and it requires some considerable planning.

WHAT YOU NEED BEFORE SETTING A DATE

Before you set a date, make sure that you have all of the necessities. Your employees should be well trained and ready to greet guests. Supplies should be well stocked and your budget should be in check. Now you just have to get ready for your opening day.

You need to prepare before setting a date. Following are some things you will need before setting a date for your opening in addition to proper licensing and regulations.

- Membership packets from the chamber of commerce in your area

- Budget for the grand opening

- Theme and activities

- Contact media venues for announcements and photo opportunities

- Create a press kit (fact sheet, biography, services, amenities)

- Hire a writer to write a press release

- Create an invitation list that includes neighboring businesses and local community service organizations

- Offer grand opening specials and coupons

- Develop a ribbon cutting ceremony with the chamber of commerce

You will also need to spread the word about your grand opening quickly and effectively. Consider the following quick tips to start you in the right direction.

- Make a distinction between advertisements and publicity. Advertisements are designed to sell. Publicity is nearly as effective but there has to be an element of human interest in the story rather than sales-focused communication.

- Get in contact with news departments in local television and radio stations and share your story.

- Introduce your new business to local newspapers.

- Put all of your contact information on any correspondence with the media, including your press release.

- Include the date that you want your story to appear in the paper.

- Deliver all correspondences with local media groups in person.

- Provide at least one photograph with your press release or human-interest story.

Advertising follows a different set of rules. Consider the following in your ad campaign:

- Circulate promotional items like t-shirts, mugs and hats.

- Advertise your unveiling ceremony using fliers.

- Purchase ad space in newspapers; small ones the week before and large ones the day before the grand opening.

- Invest in local television commercials.

- Create a message in the announcement column of the newspaper.

- Invest in radio spots about three days before the opening

You will put a lot of time and effort into your planning but conventional wisdom states that you only have one chance to make a first impression. Investing in your grand opening is a great way to ensure that your occasion will be memorable.

HOW TO MAKE YOUR OPENING A SPLASH

You probably have dreamed of your grand opening from the moment you conceived the idea of owning a day spa. This very important event gives you many opportunities to convey your vision and propose to your prospective clients. It is never too early to begin planning this event.

Create a mood that suits your style and philosophy. Choose a date and time that has significant meaning for you and that is convenient for your guests. Plan the opening to occur during times of high traffic. Consider your demographics when creating the time and date for the occasion.

Consider the events that will take place during the celebration. You can include a ribbon cutting ceremony. People can win door prizes including spa packages and products. A spokesperson can give a speech or tours of the facility.

Visitors can register for prizes by filling out cards with their information. This is a great opportunity to build a mailing list for future promotions. This approach is ideal because the visitors are attending the grand opening because they are interested in the spa and its services.

Think about the demographics when selecting a refreshment menu for the guests. If you are targeting a health-conscious group of people, donuts, chips and soda should not be on the list of items. Sparkling juice, flavored water and healthy snacks are viable options. Coffee is a typical favorite in many populations.

Putting this all together does take considerable time and effort but this allows you to communicate your vision and purpose to your potential clients. Remember your theme as you prepare your grand opening and the event is certain to make a great first impression.

A FEW PARTING WORDS

You can fulfill your dream of owning and operating a day spa. Begin with the demographics in your area. Continue to study the market and determine your customer base. This customer base leads you to select the appropriate services and products and it establishes the perfect location for your establishment.

Developing a theme that is beyond the ordinary requires some imagination. You probably have dreamed about how your spa will look and what kind of atmosphere it will offer your guests. This is an important aspect of the development of your business. Your theme communicates your personal style and taste and it can offer a welcoming environment for your customers.

You can get the necessary funding to ensure that you can afford to open your day spa. Investors are willing to provide funding. Traditional bank and other lending institution loans are viable options that work.

The Small Business Association can offer great loans for first-time business owners and many other specialty loans.

Your business plan is the heart of your day spa that can foster your theme concepts. Careful consideration and forethought as you develop and flesh out your plans can take your endeavor a long way. Your vision and purpose propel all of this into action. You are entering a wonderful field of vast opportunities.

<u>RESOURCES</u>

<u>http://dayspaassociation.com/index.htm</u>

<u>http://www.massageregister.com/staterequirements.asp</u>

<u>http://www.dayspamagazine.com/index.php</u>

<u>http://www.massagetherapy.com/careers/stateboards.php</u>

<u>http://www.sba.gov/</u>

<u>http://www.experienceispa.com/ISPA/</u>

www.ingramcontent.com/pod-product-compliance
Lightning Source LLC
Chambersburg PA
CBHW051218250726
48655CB00006B/2477